Fighting Cancer
with the Help of
Your Catholic Faith

Fighting Cancer
with the Help of
Your Catholic Faith

Lorene Hanley Duquin

Our Sunday Visitor Publishing Division
Our Sunday Visitor, Inc.
Huntington, Indiana 46750

Contents

Introduction

*B*efore anyone uttered the word, I knew I had cancer.

There were too many clues: The look on the technician's face after she developed the mammogram. The radiologist's assurance that it was "probably nothing," but should be biopsied. The medical secretary's evasiveness when I called about the biopsy results. "The doctor wants to talk to you himself," she hedged.

I thought I had prepared myself for the worst, but when I heard the doctor say "cancer," I felt as if I couldn't breathe. How could this happen to me?

The National Cancer Institute estimates that each year nearly 1,400,000 people are diagnosed with some form of cancer. Half of those diagnosed this year will continue to live full lives. Some will be completely cured. Others will go into remission or survive for years with improved treatments that control the disease and the symptoms.

Cancer is no longer an automatic death sentence. Still, I felt as if my life had been threatened. I began to plan the readings and the music for my funeral Mass.

It wasn't long before reality intruded; I had decisions to make. One doctor recommended a mastectomy. Another recommended a lumpectomy and radiation. A third recommended a double mastectomy — just to be sure. The choice was mine.

I had become accustomed to praying about major decisions, but prayer was suddenly difficult. Although I never would have admitted it at the time, a part of me was angry with God for allowing this to happen.

My first reaction was not to let anyone know. But, gradually, the news leaked out. Family members and friends rallied. People sent food and flowers, although no one knew what to say. It felt like a living wake. Something had died, but I was too numb to understand what had perished. I would learn later that my life, as I had known it, was over. A new life — in many ways a better life — was beginning.

A SPIRITUAL JOURNEY

Cancer set me on a journey that would lead me through physical, emotional, and spiritual pain. It was a journey with hills and valleys. Along the way, I met fascinating people and discovered God in a way that I never imagined possible. It was a journey I had not anticipated — a journey I wasn't prepared for — but, in the end, a journey I'm not sorry I experienced.

The purpose of this little book is to recreate the key parts of the spiritual journey through cancer. The path is marked by spiritual mileposts, but don't be surprised if you skip some of these mileposts and find yourself revisiting others several times. You may even find yourself taking side trips to experience things that aren't even mentioned.

> *The spiritual life is the greatest adventure in the world.*
> — DOROTHY DAY
> ∿

Each person's journey is unique. Whether you have been diagnosed with cancer or whether you are trying to understand the experiences of a family member or friend who has been diagnosed, you are welcome to come along. It's not an easy journey, but it is an enlightening one. And it will lead you into secret places in your heart, mind, and soul you might never have known existed.

Feeling the Feelings

A diagnosis of cancer brings a flood of emotions. Each person responds in his or her own way. For me, the news brought feelings of shock, disbelief, and denial. It's not unusual for newly diagnosed cancer patients to find themselves insisting, "No, this isn't true. I don't have cancer. This can't be happening!"

- You may question the biopsy results — especially if you don't feel sick or if you haven't experienced any lumps, bleeding, or other cancer warning signs.
- You may tell yourself that it was a mistake. Maybe they mixed up your chart with someone else's. Maybe the pathology report was wrong.
- You may find yourself thinking that it's just a bad dream, and everything will go back to normal tomorrow.
- You may not be able to think at all. A kind of numbness might overtake you.
- Some people experience panic. You may feel a desperate desire to run away, coupled with the sinking feeling that there's no place to go.
- You might go from doctor to doctor with the hope that someone will say it isn't true.
- Your prayer at this point may be more like pleading: "Please, God, don't let this happen to me." Or it may take on the tone of bargaining: "Lord, if you make this go away, I'll go to Mass every day!"

If you turn to your Catholic faith, you will find Jesus in the Garden of Gethsemane, praying, "Abba, Father, all things are possible to thee; remove this cup from me . . . " (Mk. 14:36).

> *Many of us spend our whole lives running from feeling with the mistaken belief that we cannot bear the pain. But you have already borne the pain. What you have not done is feel all that you are beyond the pain.*
>
> — ST. BARTHOLOMEW
>
> ∽

It may be a while before you are ready to finish the prayer of Jesus: "My Father, if this cannot pass unless I drink it, thy will be done" (Mt. 26:42).

WHEN IT STARTS TO FEEL REAL

Eventually, the reality of cancer crashes down on you as you move into the treatment phase of the disease. With your normal routines interrupted, you may feel like an alien entering a foreign world — you have appointments in places you've never visited before, myriad forms to fill out, a stream of new people asking the same questions over and over... you encounter strange new machines and equipment, and acquire a whole new vocabulary.

By this point, although you may still be in a state of shock, denial is no longer possible. Once you've chosen to accept treatment, it's difficult to deny the reality that you have cancer.

Fear and anxiety become the dominant emotions as you confront surgery, chemotherapy, radiation, or other cancer treatments. It can be fear of pain and suffering, fear of disfigurement, fear of making a wrong decision, fear of how your family will cope, fear of losing dignity and control, or just heart-pounding fear of what will happen next. Your sleep may be broken by nightmares. You may feel anxious and unable to concentrate. Your prayer at this point may become shorter and more desperate: "Lord, help me!"

In time, the raw fear will subside. But at this early stage, if you turn to your Catholic faith, you will begin to understand why Jesus sweated blood in the garden.

DEALING WITH FEAR

It's easier to dispel your fears if you take the time to learn about your disease, your treatments, and the possible outcomes. Jesus promises "... the truth will make you free" (Jn. 8:32). Knowledge can alleviate some of your fear of the unknown and help you make better decisions about your treatment.

It helps if you can talk about your fears with someone. You may want to make an appointment with a priest or spiritual director. Hospital chaplains can be a tremendous help at this stage of the journey.

Finding a Spiritual Director

A spiritual director is a person who has been trained to listen and help discern the movement of the Holy Spirit in your life. Spiritual direction has been part of the Catholic tradition for centuries, but only recently have increasing numbers of laypeople discovered that it is a good way to grow closer to God. To find a spiritual director, you can get referrals from friends, your pastor, the hospital chaplain, a local retreat house, the vocation director in your diocese, or the formation directors of religious communities. For additional information, contact Spiritual Directors International at 425-455-1565, or visit their Web site at www.sdiworld.org.

It's also a good idea to talk directly to God about your feelings. Jesus says, "Come to me, all who labor and are heavy laden, and I will give you rest" (Mt. 11:28). St. Peter advises: "Cast all your anxieties on him, for he cares about you" (1 Pet. 5:7).

Talking to God when you are anxious and afraid is one of the best kinds of prayer, because it comes straight from your heart. If you find this kind of prayer difficult, try writing your feelings in a spiritual journal, as if you were writing letters to God.

If that doesn't work, look for other ways to vent your emotions. One of the greatest pitfalls is to unintentionally release your anger or frustration toward family members, friends, your doctor, or the health care workers who are trying to help you. Instead, try going for walks or engaging in some kind of physical exercise. Take a bath, listen to quiet music, sit in front of a fireplace, watch the waves roll onto the beach, or gaze at the clouds drifting through the sky.

> *You need not cry very loud. God is nearer to us than we think.*
>
> — BROTHER LAWRENCE

Crying is a powerful way to release emotional tension. Some saints talk about "the gift of tears," and they may be right. Modern researchers have discovered that deeply emotional tears contain an enzyme that triggers the release of harmful toxins that build up in your body in times of stress. Crying strengthens your immune system.

I remember being afraid to cry because I thought once I started I would never stop. I also found myself fighting back tears when I was in public or when family members or friends were around. After a while, as the tension continued to build inside of me, I began to set aside "crying times" when I was taking a shower or driving in the car, and at night, when everyone else was sleeping and I was alone with God.

THE SACRAMENT OF THE SICK

At this early stage of your journey, it's a good idea to receive the Sacrament of the Sick. The *Catechism of the Catholic Church* assures us that the grace of this sacrament is "one of strengthening, peace, and courage to overcome the difficulties that go with the condition of serious illness."

The Sacrament of the Sick can be administered to you privately by a priest, in a small gathering with family members, or in a communal celebration at your parish. Your head and hands will be anointed with blessed oil as the priest says, "Through this holy anointing, may the Lord in His love and mercy help you with the grace of the Holy Spirit. May the Lord, who frees you from sin, save you and raise you up."

Is any among you sick? Let him call for the elders of the Church, and let them pray over him, anointing him with oil in the name of the Lord...

— JAS. 5:14

This anointing with holy oil gives you the grace of comfort. It offers spiritual strength. It instills in you a deeper trust in God. You can receive this sacrament again any time you face another surgery, or if your cancer progresses.

A good prayer for this stage of the journey is attributed to Pope John XXIII:

Every day I need you, Lord, but this day especially I need some extra strength to face whatever is to be. . . . This day more than any other day I need to feel You near, to fortify my courage and to overcome my fear. By myself, I cannot meet the challenge of the hour. There are times when human creatures need a higher Power to help them bear what must be borne. And so, dear Lord, I pray, that you will hold on to my trembling hand and be with me today.

QUESTIONS FOR REFLECTION

1. How did you feel when you learned you were diagnosed with cancer?
2. As you learned about your treatment, what were your greatest fears?
3. How did your faith help you through this early stage of the journey?

Asking the Ultimate Questions

*I*n the midst of your emotional whirlwind, cancer forces you to ask existential questions that most people avoid in their daily lives:

- Who am I?
- Why am I here?
- Why is this to happening to me?

> *Adversity introduces you to yourself.*
>
> — ANONYMOUS
>
> ~

These are the kinds of questions that you wrestle with in the deepest part of your soul. They are questions without clear answers that can start you on your journey toward inner peace, or divert you on a pathway into doubts and self-pity. This is one of the most important stages that you will face on your journey. You can allow the questions to move you into the light of faith, or you can allow the questions to bury you in the darkness of despair.

If you turn to your Catholic beliefs, you will find some answers.

To the question, "Who am I?" — you will be reminded that you are a child of God.

To the question, "Why am I here?" — you will recall that you were created to love and serve God and to be happy with Him in heaven.

But these simple answers are a mere introduction into the mystery of what it means to be a child of God, and the ultimate purpose of this life and the next. Cancer is your invitation to weigh these mysteries in the depths of your being. Your attitudes toward God, yourself, and others, your deepest beliefs, your values, and your priorities in life will all come under scrutiny. You may find that things you used to think were important will begin to take a lesser role in your life. Likewise, things that you always took for granted will increase in importance.

> *Seek not to understand that you may believe, but believe that you may understand.*
>
> — ST. AUGUSTINE
>
> ~

It's a process that will continue throughout your struggle with cancer. Just when you think you've found an answer, new questions will arise. At some point on this journey, you will face the most difficult question of all: "Why is this happening to me?"

WHY ME?

For some, the answer will be painfully obvious. If you had a history of smoking or lifestyle choices that caused your cancer, you may wrestle with guilt or regret. Another cancer patient told me that it brought her back to the Sacrament of Reconciliation, where she sobbed, "I did this to myself, and now I am so sorry." There was no reprimand, only a lifting of guilt, the permission to forgive herself, and the strong reassurance that God would be with her in the days ahead.

Be patient toward all that is unsolved within you and try to love the questions. The point is to live everything. Do not seek answers that cannot be lived, but love the questions, and perhaps without knowing it you will live your way into the answers.

— RAINER MARIA RILKE

If there was a genetic or environmental factor that caused your cancer, you may feel anger or outrage at the unfairness of it all. You may feel like an innocent victim, and you may worry about family members being subjected to the same fate.

You may feel angry with God for allowing this to happen. It may be hard to imagine at this early point, but you will have the opportunity to transform your feelings of rage into anger at the *disease*, then use that anger to fight the cancer cells in your body.

Knowing the physical cause of your cancer gives you something that you can point to, someplace where you can lay the blame. For many people, however, there is no clear-cut reason for the disease. For some reason, certain cells have become aggressive and destructive, and you may never know why.

You might begin to speculate: Maybe it is just a fluke of nature. Maybe it is a curse. A twist of fate? Bad luck? Some kind of punishment? When your questions take you down that path, you come face-to-face with the question: How could God allow this to happen?

Someone suggested to me that if God has given us free will to choose good or evil, maybe that freedom has also been extended to the cells in our bodies. The idea shook me to the core of myself. If I could no longer trust my body, my own cells, what could I trust? Is everything out of control? I began to wonder if I could trust God.

One woman told me that her only prayer at this stage was an agonizing, "Why? Why? Why?"

THE EXPERIENCE OF JOB

If you turn to Scripture, you will find Job wrestling with some of these same questions as he goes over every detail of his life to find some reason for his suffering. Like Job, you may insist that you have done nothing to cause cancer. Like Job, you may find yourself crying out, ". . . let the Almighty answer me!" (Job 31:35). And, like Job, you will discover that God doesn't answer the question "why." Instead, God asks Job a series of questions that make Job see the extent of God's power in all of creation.

Lord, I do not ask that I never be afflicted, but only that you never abandon me in affliction.

— ST. BERNADETTE SOUBIROUS

"I have uttered what I did not understand," Job finally admits, "things too wonderful for me, which I did not know" (Job 42:3).

In the end, God restored Job's life and prosperity. But the greatest gift Job received was a closer relationship with the Lord, and the realization that the Lord was present to him in his time of need. God remained close to Job as he wrestled with his questions about the mystery of suffering, and even though the Lord did not answer Job's questions directly, He graced Job with His presence.

As I wrestled with all of this, a wise priest assured me that someday, I would understand my diagnosis of cancer in a different light — perhaps even from God's perspective — but I wasn't yet far enough along on the journey. I had, however, reached a point where I could make a choice: I could believe that cancer was a curse, or I could believe that cancer was, in some strange way, a blessing I did not fully understand. If I chose to see cancer as a curse, I would remain where I was on the path, and I would fall into self-pity and despair. If I chose to believe that something good would come from this adversity and God would transform my life, then I

Ask, and it will be given you; seek, and you will find; knock, and it will be opened to you.

— LK. 11:9

would move a little further on the journey toward inner peace. The choice was mine. The choice is yours.

❧ QUESTIONS FOR REFLECTION ❧

1. How did you struggle with the "why" questions?
2. How has your diagnosis affected your relationship with God?
3. Do you see cancer as a curse, or as some kind of strange blessing that you don't understand yet?

Facing Your Own Death

*M*odern society considers death a horrible catastrophe that intrudes upon our sense of youthfulness, optimism, and self-sufficiency. No one wants to think about death. No one wants to talk about it. But as Catholics we are told, "Every illness can make us glimpse death" (*CCC*, 1500).

After my diagnosis, I began to think a lot about my funeral.

- Who would say the Mass?
- What readings and music would I choose?
- Who would carry my casket into the church?
- Who would bring up the gifts?
- How would I be remembered?

Before long, deeper questions emerged.

- What would happen to me after I died?
- Could I trust the Catholic belief that there would be everlasting life?
- Or, would I give in to nagging doubts that after death there is nothing but darkness and aloneness?

I took comfort in the words of the late Cardinal Basil Hume, O.S.B., who wrote, "As we approach the last bit of the journey there are days when we fear that we face an unknown, unpredictable, uncertain future. That is a common experience." He went on to say that as time goes on, we let go of those fears and we travel through the darkness into the light of God's love. He was convinced that death was the "way which leads us to the vision of God."

Our Catholic faith tells us that the death of Jesus is a model for our own death. Many people find comfort in meditating on the image of a crucifix and the words of Jesus, "Father, into your hands I commit my Spirit" (Lk.

> *I consider that the sufferings of this present time are not worth comparing with the glory that is to be revealed to us.*
>
> — ROM. 8:18
>
> ∽

> *Dying is not extraneous to life; it is part of the mystery.*
> *And you do not understand life until you stand under death.*
>
> — RICHARD ROHR
>
> ❧

23:46), which assure us of the nearness of God at the moment of Jesus' death.

The catechism teaches that death has been "transformed by Christ," who turned "the curse of death into a blessing" (*CCC,* 1009). Jesus holds the promise of eternal life through His death and resurrection.

BEFRIENDING DEATH

When Cardinal Joseph Bernardin was dying from pancreatic cancer, spiritual writer Henri Nouwen advised the cardinal to befriend death. "People of faith, who believe death is the transition from this life to life eternal, should see it as a friend," Nouwen explained.

Saints have often urged that facing our own death will diminish our fear and give us a deeper appreciation for life and the many gifts of God that we tend to take for granted.

- The Rule of St. Benedict states, "Keep death daily before your eyes."
- St. Ignatius of Loyola encouraged people to meditate on their own death as a way of discerning the essential from the non-essential in life.
- St. Philip Neri said the best way to prepare for death is to live each day as if it were your last.
- St. Alphonsus Liguori insisted that reflecting upon death leads to wisdom and opens our souls to the graces needed to live a good life in whatever time we have left.

Don't be surprised if your prayers and meditations on death make you begin to see everything from a different perspective.

- Facing death brings to the forefront all of the joys of life, but it also surfaces the disappointments, sorrows, sins, and regrets about things you haven't yet been able to do. If you find yourself struggling with all of this, it's a good idea to make an appointment with a priest or spiritual director. The Sacrament of Reconciliation can get rid of any useless guilt you might feel and bring you to a deeper level of peace.

> *If only we could make people understand that we come from God and that we have to go back to him!*
>
> — BLESSED MOTHER TERESA OF CALCUTTA
>
> ~

- Facing death helps you sort out your priorities in terms of what is really important. It helps you to rid yourself of things that are unimportant and focus on what is closest to your heart. It encourages you to tackle projects you always wanted to accomplish, and to finish things you have left undone.

- Facing death makes you realize each moment is precious. It encourages you to let go of the past, set aside anxiety about the future, and live to the fullest in the present moment.

- Facing death gives you a deeper understanding of what it means to love and to be loved.

- Facing death instills in you a desire to forgive people who have hurt you and to seek the forgiveness of people you have hurt.

- Facing death strengthens your faith as you begin to see death as a process of transition from one state of being to another.

- Facing death allows you to embrace life and develop a deep appreciation for each new day. You may begin to feel more alive than you ever felt before.

- Facing death also brings some serious responsibilities. As a Catholic, it is important for you to complete an advance directive stating what kind of medical care you want, or do not want, in the event you become physically or mentally unable to state your preferences. If you don't put into writing your wishes regarding pain medications, life support, resuscitation, feeding tubes, and other emergency medical procedures, someone else will make these decisions for you, and those decisions may not be in line with your desires or your religious beliefs.

It's also important to talk to someone about the details of your death. It could be a family member, a friend, a priest, a spiritual director, or someone else that you trust. These are the things that you should put into writing:

> *Courage is almost a contradiction in terms. It means a strong desire to live taking the form of readiness to die.*
>
> — G. K. CHESTERTON
>
> ᘒ

- Would you prefer to die at home, in a hospice, or in a hospital?
- After you die, how would you like your body to be cared for, and by whom?
- Do you want your body to be autopsied?
- Do you want to donate any organs that can be salvaged?
- Do you want to plan the details of your funeral?
- Do you want to be buried or cremated?
- Do you want your remains laid to rest in a Catholic cemetery?
- How do you want to be remembered? Is there some legacy that you want to leave?

Now is also the time to take care of the temporal aspects of your life. Do you have a will? Are your personal papers and belongings in order?

It's not easy to face your own mortality. You may find that you can cope with all of this only in small doses. But in time you will discover that, while facing your own death takes courage, it will lead to a new sense of freedom and a growing sense of peace. Handling death well is one of the surest signs that we have lived a good life.

A powerful prayer for this stage of your journey is the *Anima Christi*:

Soul of Christ, sanctify me.
Body of Christ, save me.
Blood of Christ, inebriate me.
Water from Christ's side, wash me.
Passion of Christ, strengthen me.
O good Jesus, hear me.
Within Thy wounds hide me.
Suffer me not to be separated from Thee.
From the malicious enemy, defend me.
In the hour of my death, call me.
And bid me come unto Thee,

That I may praise Thee with Thy saints
And with Thy angels
Forever and ever,
Amen.

∾ QUESTIONS FOR REFLECTION ∾

1. In what ways have you reflected upon your own death?
2. In what ways have you prepared for your death?
3. How has the reality of death impacted your faith and your relationship with God?

Dealing with Other People

Shortly after I was diagnosed, I received a bouquet of roses from a woman I had never met. She was a friend of a friend, and she had survived breast cancer. She sent the flowers with a little note assuring me of her prayers and saying I could call her if I wanted to talk, but if not, that was okay, too.

Don't expect that kind of sensitivity from everybody.

- Some people avoid you, probably because they don't know what to say or do, and it's easier to stay away.
- Some people act strangely around you because your illness makes them feel vulnerable. You can almost see them thinking, "If it could happen to him/her, it could happen to me!"
- Some people tell you stories about family members or friends who have had cancer. Sometimes, these stories do not have happy endings.
- Some people ask you embarrassing questions about your diagnosis.
- Some people focus on trying to figure out what caused your cancer.

> *Real friends are those rare people who ask how you are and then wait to hear the answer.*
>
> — ANONYMOUS
>
> ~

Don't let yourself become upset by other people's behavior. There are far more important ways for you to use your energy. In most cases, these people mean no harm. When confronted with insensitivity, you can find real comfort in the prayer of Jesus, "Father, forgive them; for they know not what they do" (Lk. 23:34).

WHEN HELPERS HURT

There are some people whose behavior can be hazardous to your well-being. These are the people who harass you with unsolicited advice about what doctor to choose, what to eat, what vitamins to take, and what treatments to undergo or to avoid.

> *A faithful friend is a sturdy shelter.*
>
> — SIR. 6:14
>
>

Don't waste your time or energy on someone who undermines your morale or treatment. If you look at Scripture, you'll find that when Jesus told the apostles that His mission would lead to suffering and death, Peter was appalled and blurted out, "God forbid, Lord! No such thing shall ever happen to you" (Mt. 16:22).

Jesus would not be deterred from what He knew was God's will. He accused Peter of being a "hindrance to me" (Mt. 16:23). Likewise, you may have to take a firm stand against people who become a hindrance to you.

FIND A GOOD SUPPORT SYSTEM

Surround yourself with people who will support you through this difficult time.

- Look for people who are good listeners. They don't question you or try to change the way you're feeling. They just listen.
- Look for people who really want to help. They run errands, do the shopping, and bring casseroles for dinner. They might offer to drive you to treatments. If they're really good friends, they might clean your house, cut your lawn, or take over household chores.
- Look for people who cheer you up. They make you laugh. They offer a diversion and let you forget about cancer for a while. They may come and watch a movie with you or take you out for lunch. Sometimes, just their presence is enough to brighten your day.

DEALING WITH FAMILY MEMBERS

You might expect that the most helpful people will be your family members, but that isn't always the case. Throughout your illness, the people closest to you will experience some of the same emotional and spiritual turmoil that you experience. They will find themselves asking the same existential questions. As they face the possibility of your death, they will confront their own mortality. You are the one who was diagnosed with cancer, but they are suffering, too.

Serious illness changes relationships — sometimes for better, sometimes for worse — and there doesn't seem to be any accurate way of predicting how family members will deal with your diagnosis. You may have expectations of them that they are unable or unwilling to meet. Likewise, they may have expectations of you that seem to be beyond your physical or emotional capabilities. Some will try to put up a positive front with lots of smiles and encouragement. Others will retreat silently into their own fears. In time, resentments on both sides can fester.

A LONELY DISEASE

While I was undergoing treatment, a technician told me that her mother-in-law was dying from cancer, and she was the only person in the family who would talk to her about it. "Cancer is a lonely disease," her mother-in-law admitted, "because it can isolate you emotionally from the people who are closest to you."

I was in the opposite situation. I was the one who didn't want to talk about it. I needed solitude in order to come to grips with my diagnosis, but I drew too far into myself. I came dangerously close to isolating myself. A priest suggested that I try to write about my feelings to my husband and children.

"This has been a very difficult time and I've been pretty self-absorbed," I finally admitted in writing. "It's hard for me to think of myself in terms of being a cancer patient. The reality of having cancer hits me like a punch in the stomach. There are a lot of fears connected to all of this. I am trying to be as normal as possible, but I am beginning to see that it isn't always possible. I know that I have been drawn inside of myself a lot more lately. I'm beginning to think that it's a part of this illness that involves a 'coming to grips with' on a psychological, emotional, and spiritual level. I'm sorry if I've hurt you as a result of this. It's not intentional. I understand that this has

---

When we honestly ask ourselves which persons in our lives mean the most to us, we often find that it is those who, instead of giving advice, solutions, or cures, have chosen rather to share our pain and touch our wounds with a warm and tender hand. The friend who can be silent with us in a moment of despair or confusion, who can stay with us in an hour of grief and bereavement, who can tolerate not knowing, not curing, not healing and face with us the reality of our powerlessness, that is a friend who cares.

— HENRI NOUWEN

been a very difficult time for you, too. It's like the rug has been pulled out from the foundation of our lives and everything is askew. I wish that I could put it all together again and that things could go back to normal, but I don't know if that is possible."

It opened the lines of communication. My husband and children admitted how difficult it was for them. They were frightened. They didn't know what to say or do.

I learned a few things about myself, too.

- I didn't want to be a burden to anyone, so it was very difficult for me to accept help from other people. When I realized how much the people closest to me wanted to help, and how frustrated they were at not knowing what to do, I learned to try to think of things they could do that would be a real comfort to me.
- I became more conscious of trying to let people know when I felt weak or exhausted, so they would understand why I was retreating to my room to rest.
- I learned that I couldn't dictate how another person was going to act or react. I could only communicate what I was thinking or feeling, and I could try to listen to what the other person was saying. But I could not control the outcome. Some things just had to unfold in their own way.
- I learned that one of the best things that I could do for myself and for other people was to ask them to pray for me.

A prayer that might help you at this stage of the journey is the Serenity Prayer:

*Lord, grant me the serenity
To accept the things I cannot change,
The courage to change the things I can,
And the wisdom to know the difference.*

∾ QUESTIONS FOR REFLECTION ∾

1. What kinds of positive and negative experiences have you encountered with other people?
2. How is your family dealing with your diagnosis?
3. Who are the people who have helped you the most?

Giving Up Control

*M*ost of us operate under the illusion that we have control over our lives; cancer shatters that illusion. It pushes us out of our safe little existence into a new world filled with uncertainty. It forces us to accept the fact that we are vulnerable. It forces us to admit we do not know what tomorrow will bring. It forces us to face our own powerlessness.

The first indication that my life was not under my control was the overwhelming feeling that my body had betrayed me. My cells were multiplying abnormally. I was not in control.

Lack of control continued to manifest itself in other ways. It happened as I was being wheeled into the operating room. I knew that for the next few hours I would be unconscious, and my life would be in the hands of other people. I was not in control.

In the weeks after the surgery, pain and tiredness destroyed my daily routine. I couldn't do some of the things that I wanted to do. I had to accept my own limitations. I was not in control.

Just as I was beginning to feel stronger and life seemed to be getting back to normal, daily radiation treatments began for a six-week period. I tried to schedule the sessions in the early afternoon so I could still work in

My Lord and God, I have no idea where I am going. I do not see the road ahead of me. I cannot know for certain where it will end. Nor do I really know myself, and the fact that I think that I am following your will does not mean that I am actually doing so. But I believe that the desire to please you does in fact please you. And I hope I have that desire in all that I am doing. I hope that I will never do anything apart from that desire. And I know that if I do this you will lead me by the right road though I may know nothing about it.

— THOMAS MERTON

∾

And which of you by being anxious can add one cubit to his span of life?

— MT. 6:27

∽

the mornings, but halfway through the treatments, deep fatigue set in. I couldn't concentrate. I couldn't work. Once again, I felt as if my life had spun out of my control.

Chemotherapy, nausea, hair loss, and other side effects continue this stressful process. Your life is changing, and there is nothing you can do to stop it. You can try to fight it, but you'll find yourself getting frustrated every time your plans are disrupted. It's much better if you can begin to let go.

WHAT TO LEAVE BEHIND

Let go of any remnants of denial. Cancer has become a part of your life and there's no escape. Letting go means accepting the fact that you have cancer.

- Let go of your personal agenda. Your physical limitations may prevent you from doing what you used to do. Letting go means finding joy and satisfaction in whatever things you can accomplish.
- Let go of unrealistic expectations. You begin to see that all of your dreams for the future may not come true. Letting go means finding a new appreciation of what is happening in the present moment. The past is gone, and the future is unknown. The only place where you will find God is in the present moment.
- Let go of superficiality. Your outward appearance will probably change because of surgery, fatigue, weight gain or loss, and other side effects. Letting go means that you come to understand that what you look like on the outside is not the real you. It's the person you are on the inside that counts.
- Let go of self-sufficiency. You may find that you are not as independent as you used to be. Letting go means learning how to ask other people for help.
- Let go of worry. You can't change or control anything with worry. It only creates more tension in you and the people around you. Letting go means placing everything in God's hands and accepting the fact that whatever is going to happen will happen, whether you worry about it or not.

THE PROCESS OF LETTING GO

It should be understood at this point that "letting go" does *not* mean you stop trying to fight the disease. It doesn't mean you give up on life. It means that you empty yourself of everything that is not important, and in the process of emptying yourself, you allow God to fill the empty spaces of your being.

When Fr. Richard John Neuhaus was undergoing treatment for cancer, he recalled that the process of letting go left him on the edge of tears. "Not in sadness," he said. "Not at all. But in a kind of amazement that this had happened to me, and maybe I was going to die and maybe I was going to live, and it was all quite out of my control. That was it, I think: I was not in charge, and it was both strange and very good not to be in charge."

If you turn to your Catholic faith, you will discover that letting go is the essence of authentic spirituality. Once you begin to let go, you can focus the energy you used to spend trying to control everything into a more positive direction toward the things that are really important. It's a process of leaning how to place your trust in God. It is only when we let go of our personal agenda and surrender to the will of God that we learn how to live. Jesus tells us, "For whoever would save his life will lose it, and whoever loses his life for my sake will find it" (Mt. 16:25).

> *We cannot enjoy true peace unless we submit to God's will.*
>
> — JEAN-PIERRE DE CAUSSADE

Surrender to the will of God is not easy. You may find that you have to consciously surrender every day of your life. St. Ignatius of Loyola wrote a prayer that captures the essence of that surrender:

> *Take, O Lord, and receive my entire liberty, my memory, my understanding and my whole will. All that I am and all that I possess You have given me: I surrender it all to You to be disposed of according to Your will. Give me only Your love and Your grace; with these I will be rich enough, and will desire nothing more.*

THE PATH TO SAINTHOOD

Most people don't take sainthood seriously. They idealize saints; they put them safely on a pedestal where they can admire them; but they don't really believe that an "ordinary person" like them could ever become a saint. Cancer is one of those extraordinary things that opens a special pathway toward sainthood, but it's your choice whether or not you want to take that path . . . a path of surrender to the will of God.

If God allows you to suffer much, it is a sign that he certainly intends to make you a saint.

— ST. IGNATIUS OF LOYOLA

When I was in the midst of struggling with all of this, a priest used the analogy of a vineyard to explain the process. When the grapes are ripe, they are plucked from the vines and thrown into a large vat, where they are crushed. That's what had happened to me. I had been crushed by cancer. I had been stripped of my life as it had been before. I was crushed and fermenting, but I had a choice: I could come out of this process as wine, or I could come out of this process as vinegar. I could come out of it holier and closer to God, or I could come out of it bitter and closer to despair. I decided that I wanted to be wine. It's a choice that we all have to make.

QUESTIONS FOR REFLECTION

1. What are some of the things that you have to "let go"?
2. What do you think God's will is for you during this time of your life?
3. Are you ready to begin thinking of yourself on the path toward sainthood?

Discovering New Ways to Pray

I was still recovering from my cancer treatments when my daughter's 26-year-old boyfriend was diagnosed with malignant melanoma. Because I had some free time, I was the one who accompanied Michael to most of his doctor's appointments and hospital treatments. Michael had received very little spiritual formation as a child. He had a lot of questions about God. He wanted to know how to pray.

> *When you come before the Lord, talk to him if you can; if you can't, just stay there, let yourself be seen, and don't try too hard to do anything else*
>
> — ST. FRANCIS DE SALES
>
> ∾

I tried to explain that prayer is not just repeating words or even reading words. It is communication with God on a very intimate level. It begins with a deep desire to seek God and develops into a loving relationship where we give ourselves to God. Then we respond to God as He makes himself known to us. Prayer calms our fear, displaces worry, and reduces stress. Prayer changes us. It changes our outlook on our problems.

My experience of cancer had changed the way I prayed, and now this new experience with Michael was allowing me to share with him some of the things I had learned on my journey.

THE POWER OF PRAYER

While prayer is important for your spiritual well being, medical researchers are now discovering that prayer also plays a role in physical healing. Recent studies show that faith in God and prayer:

- Helps to lower blood pressure,
- Strengthens the immune system,
- Reduces anxiety, discomfort, and sense of isolation,
- Shortens hospital stays,
- Increases the quality of life and the ability to adjust to cancer treatments, and

> *Likewise the Spirit helps us in our weakness; for we do not know how to pray as we ought, but the Spirit himself intercedes for us with sighs too deep for words. And he who searches the hearts of men knows what is the mind of the Spirit, because the Spirit intercedes for the saints according to the will of God.*
>
> — ROM. 8:26-27

- Improves health outcomes.

Other studies conclude that patients who pray seem happier, suffer less from depression, and are better able to cope with their health challenges. There are even studies that suggest people who are prayed for by others tend to recover more quickly. While medical professionals try to discover the reasons for the power of prayer, as Catholics we can simply take it as a matter of faith. Look through the Gospels and you'll see that almost every time Jesus healed someone, He said, "Your faith has healed you" or "Your faith has saved you." St. Paul tells us that God "rewards those who seek him" (Heb. 11:6). He also advises us to "pray constantly" (1 Thess. 5:17).

CATHOLIC FORMS OF PRAYER

As Catholics, we believe that the Eucharist is our primary source of healing because each time we take communion, we receive the real presence of Christ, "body and blood, soul and divinity," into our own bodies. Jesus becomes one with us.

When you are unable to receive Communion, you can make a Spiritual Communion by praying:

My Jesus, I love you above all things, and I long for You in my soul.
Come into my heart spiritually and never let me be separated from You.

At some point on your journey through cancer, you might want to take the opportunity to attend a special Healing Mass. During the Mass, the intentions of the participants are prayed for in a special way. After the Mass, you can approach the altar where a priest, or teams of laypeople, will pray over you. Many people find this a powerful experience of prayer that can bring spiritual, if not physical, healing.

Another source of consolation and strength to many cancer patients is Eucharistic Adoration, which places you in the presence of the Lord. One cancer patient called it her special form of "radiation" therapy, because she could feel the rays of love coming to her from the Blessed Sacrament.

> *Prayer enlarges the heart until it is capable of containing God's gift of Himself.*
>
> — BLESSED MOTHER TERESA OF CALCUTTA

PRAYING WITH THE PSALMS

The book of Psalms is another source of spiritual and emotional support in times of illness. In the psalms, you will find a complete range of human needs and emotions. The psalms are like conversations with God in which you can join the psalmist in pouring out your deepest feelings.

Throughout the psalms there are many references to "enemies." While praying the psalms, keep in mind that your enemies are cancer cells. Use the psalms as another way of asking God to destroy those cells.

Here are some verses from the psalms that you might find helpful in your journey through cancer:

- When times are hard: Psalms 138, 94,18, 69, and 86.
- When you want God's protection: Psalms 70, 27, 91, and 84.
- When you want God's guidance: Psalms 16, 25, 121, and 146.
- When you need to depend on God: Psalms 3, 30, 62, and 71.
- When it feels like God isn't there: Psalms 22, 13, 63, and 42.
- When you want to thank God: Psalms 41, 93, and 103.
- When you want to praise God: Psalms 92, 100, 150, and 113.

TURNING VISUALIZATIONS INTO PRAYER

It's usually not long after your diagnosis that someone will tell you about visualizations in which you imagine that your cancer cells are being attacked by an army of white blood cells that destroy the cancer and force it out of your body. Studies show that visualizations have positive results with cancer patients. What I discovered is that you can also turn your visualizations into a prayer.

Begin by closing your eyes and totally relaxing your body. Imagine that you are in a fountain of God's love. Feel the water come down on you.

Maybe it is warm and soothing, or maybe it is cool and refreshing. Imagine that God is cleansing you with His love. Ask God to wash away any guilt, anger, resentment, tension, or pain that you might be experiencing. Now imagine that you are filling your cupped hands with water from the fountain and drink the water. Imagine God's love flowing through your body and flushing out the cancer cells.

> The function of prayer is not to influence God, but rather to change the nature of the one who prays.
>
> — SÖREN KIERKEGAARD
>
> ◡

Turning your visualizations into prayer is a form of meditation. The catechism tells us that meditation is a form of mental prayer that "engages thought, imagination, emotion, and desire . . . in order to deepen our convictions of faith, prompt the conversion of our heart, and strengthen our will to follow Christ" (*CCC*, 2708).

As you become more experienced in this form of prayer, you can change the images that you use in your meditation by placing yourself in the scene of a Scripture passage. You might imagine that you are present when Jesus heals someone, or standing at the foot of the cross with Our Lady.

The Rosary is another form of meditative prayer. The repetition of the Hail Marys keeps your mind focused while you meditate on the mysteries of the life of Christ.

PRAYING IN THE PRESENCE OF GOD

Contemplation is a form of prayer that can help you calm your mind, broaden your spiritual horizons, and transcend the physical limitations cancer has imposed upon you. In meditation, you use your mind and your imagination to think about God; in contemplation, you free yourself from all thoughts and simply place yourself in the presence of God.

To begin, sit comfortably with your palms in an open position on your lap. Take a few deep breaths and feel the air move in and out of your lungs. Close your eyes and empty your mind by quietly repeating a word or phrase as a kind of mantra. Some people use the Jesus prayer: "Lord Jesus Christ, Son of God, have mercy on me, a sinner." Others shorten it to, "Jesus, mercy," or simply repeat the word "Jesus." If you find your mind wandering, keep bringing it back with your breathing and your simple mantra.

St. Peregrine, Patron Saint of Cancer Patients

St. Peregrine was born in Forli, Italy around 1265 — a time when the city was in turmoil because of anti-papal political activity, and neither the Mass nor the sacraments could be celebrated. St. Philip Benizi, the prior of the Servants of Mary, went to Forli to preach repentance. The young Peregrine was so involved in the politics of the day that he heckled Philip during his talks. One day, in a moment of extreme emotion, he struck Philip; horrified by that violent act, Peregrine turned his life around and started to do good works. Eventually, he joined the Servants of Mary and dedicated himself to the sick, the poor, and the people on the edges of society.

At age 60, he developed an open, running sore on his leg that was diagnosed as cancer. Surgery was scheduled to amputate his leg. However, the night before the operation, while praying intently before a crucifix, he saw the crucified Christ come down from the cross and touch his cancerous leg. When the vision ended, Peregrine was completely healed. St. Peregrine lived another 20 years, to age 80. He is the patron saint of those who suffer from cancer.

Prayer to St. Peregrine

O great St. Peregrine, you have been called "The Mighty," "The Wonder-Worker," because of the numerous miracles which you have obtained from God for those who have had recourse to you. For so many years you bore in your own flesh this cancerous disease that destroys the very fiber of our being. You had recourse to the source of all grace when the power of man could do no more. You were favored with the vision of Jesus coming down from His Cross to heal your affliction. Ask, of God and Our Lady, the cure of the sick whom we entrust to you.

(Pause here and silently include your own name and any other people for whom you are praying)

Aided in this way by your powerful intercession, we shall sing to God, now and for all eternity, a song of gratitude for His great goodness and mercy. Amen.

How great is the power of Prayer!

— ST. THÉRÈSE
OF LISIEUX

It is in this prayer of silence that you begin to feel God's presence in a special way. You begin to know that you are not alone in your battle with cancer. You will find that you become calmer, more loving, and more positive in your outlook — even when things are not going well. It's all part of the healing power of prayer.

St. Teresa of Ávila captured the essence of prayer when she wrote:

Let nothing disturb you;
Let nothing dismay you.
All things pass;
God never changes.
Patience attains all that it strives for.
He who has God finds he lacks nothing.
God alone suffices.

QUESTIONS FOR REFLECTION

1. What kinds of prayer have helped you in your battle with cancer?
2. What images do you use in visualizations or meditations?
3. Can you share some experiences of being touched by God?

Dealing with Pain

*B*efore my first surgery, the operating room nurse lifted two side panels on either side of the operating table. Then she gently extended my arms and strapped them to the panels. "It's like you're being crucified," she said.

Cancer is a kind of crucifixion, and physical pain is part of what you will experience. In the process, you will learn that pain can be a great teacher. It can teach you important lessons about God, yourself, and others. Suffering can bring you to a greater degree of holiness. It all depends on how you deal with your pain.

The first step is to accept the fact that pain exists. Pain is part of the human condition. You can't escape pain by denying it. And, even with the most powerful pain medications, you can't always avoid it.

A better approach is to try to understand your pain and what is causing it. You may be surprised to learn that the intensity of physical pain can be influenced by emotions such as anxiety, tension or fear.

> *By suffering for us He not only provided us with an example for our imitation, He blazed a trail, and if we follow it, life and death are made holy and take on a new meaning.*
>
> — *GAUDIUM ET SPES*
>
> ∾

I was afraid of pain. I could feel myself tense up hours before even the simplest of tests. Looking back, I can see that my fear of pain was always worse than any of the physical pain that I actually experienced.

WHEN PRAYER IS IMPOSSIBLE

It's not always easy to pray when you are in pain: there are too many distractions, and discomfort leaves you unable to concentrate. Even so, there was one prayer that I could use at any time and in any place, no matter how much pain I was experiencing: I simply turned my breathing into a prayer.

The "breathing prayer" is a prayer of the imagination in which you picture that you are breathing in God's love as you inhale, then exhaling any tension you feel. Breathe in God's love, and exhale fear of pain. Breathe in

> *We are afflicted in every way, but not crushed; perplexed, but not driven to despair, persecuted, but not forsaken; struck down, but not destroyed; always carrying in the body the death of Jesus, so that the life of Jesus may also be manifested in our bodies.*
>
> — 2 COR. 4: 8-10

God's love, and exhale any discomfort you feel. As you breathe in, you imagine that God's love is flowing through you to every part of your body. As you exhale, you let go of anything that is not of God.

The more you practice this prayer, the more you begin to feel God's presence, and the easier it is to deal with pain and discomfort. I used this prayer whenever I had painful tests, needle pricks, examinations that required poking or prodding, radiation treatments, and other procedures that caused anxiety or discomfort. The prayer calmed me. It also invited God into the situation, and it seemed as if the doctors, nurses, and technicians were calmer, too.

OTHER KINDS OF PAIN

In some ways, physical pain is the easiest pain to endure because it can usually be controlled with medications. Don't suffer needlessly if there is a way of alleviating your pain. Managing your pain takes patience and good communication skills. You have to let your doctor know about what kind of discomfort you feel, the intensity of the pain, and whatever side effects you experience from the pain medications.

A more difficult kind of pain to face is the emotional and spiritual pain that comes with cancer. If you turn to the Gospel accounts of Jesus' passion, you will see that in addition to the immense physical pain of the crucifixion, He suffered the pains of loss and loneliness, rejection by His friends, public ridicule, and failure in the eyes of the world.

Physical strength is measured by what we can carry; spiritual strength is measured by what we can bear.

— ANONYMOUS

Cancer can bring these kinds of suffering, too. It brings the pain of losing your hair, the pain of disfigurement, and the pain of losing bodily functions. Cancer can leave you feeling exhausted. Your ability to concentrate and make decisions can be impaired. You may have trouble sleeping. You may feel frustrated because you can't do the things you want to do.

Jesus tells us, "If any man would come after me, let him deny himself and take up his cross and follow me" (Mt. 16:24). Cancer is the cross that you are being asked to carry.

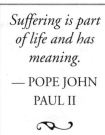

Suffering is part of life and has meaning.

— POPE JOHN PAUL II

EMBRACING THE CROSS

After Fr. Jim Willig was diagnosed with renal cell cancer that had metastasized to his lungs, he would hold onto a crucifix with the hope that God would give him the strength to carry the cross wherever it would lead. The more he clung to the cross, the more he began to change his attitude toward pain.

"Somewhere along this course, I moved beyond accepting my cross, to embracing it," he recalled. "My cross doesn't get any lighter, nor does my suffering get any easier. But as I learn to embrace my cross and believe it is the way I can become one with Jesus, the joy and peace I feel being one with Jesus is actually greater than any physical pain I feel."

OFFERING IT UP

Uniting your suffering to the suffering of Jesus makes you an active participant in the saving work of Christ. It allows you to "offer up" your pain for some greater purpose. With Jesus, and in Jesus, you can obtain the graces you need for yourself and for others.

At one point in my journey a priest asked me if I was going to "offer up" my suffering. "Yes," I told him. "I am offering it up for people who are away from the Church and struggling with faith." He smiled. "I was hoping you would offer it for priests," he replied.

His response affirmed for me that there can be purpose and power connected with pain, if you look at it from a spiritual perspective. We can "offer up" our pain by simply asking God to use our suffering for some specific intention or some person.

Just as the passion, death, and resurrection of Christ gave new meaning to suffering, uniting your suffering to the suffering of Jesus by "offering it up" can give new meaning and purpose to your pain. If God allowed the suffering of Jesus in order for something greater to hap-

I suffer much but do I suffer well? That is the important thing.

— ST. THÉRÈSE OF LISIEUX

> Pain provides an opportunity for heroism; the opportunity is seized with surprising frequency.
>
> — C. S. LEWIS
>
> ༄

pen — the salvation of all mankind — God can also bring something good out of your suffering. Uniting your pain with the pain of Christ brings you the promise of resurrection and new life.

Once you have accepted your cross, you begin to see more clearly the crosses that others carry. In time, you will discover that God is with you in the midst of your suffering and you will realize that, strange as it may seem from the "outside looking in," you *have* been blessed.

St. Paul reminds us, "For the word of the cross is folly to those who are perishing, but to us who are being saved it is the power of God" (1 Cor. 1:18).

༄ QUESTIONS FOR REFLECTION ༄

1. What kinds of pain have you experienced?
2. How do you deal with your pain?
3. How have you been able to "offer up" your pain for some greater purpose?

Overcoming Temptations

$\mathcal{A}$t one point on my journey, a friend e-mailed me a story about a man who had been asked by God to push a large rock. For years the man pushed, but the rock never moved. Recognizing an opportunity for temptation, Satan began to taunt the man by pointing out that after all that pushing, nothing had happened. The man was tempted toward hopelessness and despair. But God intervened and reminded the man that he had never been asked to move the rock, only to push it, and in the process the man's muscles had become strong and toned. There was purpose in what the man was doing, but he hadn't seen it until he understood the situation from God's perspective.

> *Everything tempts the man who fears temptation.*
> — FRENCH PROVERB
> ❧

It's sometimes difficult to see cancer from God's perspective, and that leaves us open to temptations.

RECOGNIZING TEMPTATIONS

The catechism warns that serious illnesses, like cancer, can lead to "anguish, self-absorption, sometimes even despair and revolt against God" (*CCC*, 1501). Some other temptations that cancer patients encounter include:

- Temptation toward envy when we begin to compare our lives with the experiences of people who don't have cancer.
- Temptation toward irritability when our discomfort becomes a rationale for not being nice to other people — especially those who are trying to help us.
- Temptation to constant complaining when we slip into negative attitudes that lead to criticism of both others and ourselves.
- Temptation to doubt when we forget to fix our eyes on God.
- Temptation to self-pity when we begin to feel sorry for ourselves.
- Temptation to despair when self-pity erodes our faith and our hope.

UNDERSTANDING TEMPTATIONS

Temptation is not sin, but it can lead to sin. It's important to recognize when we are being tempted. Our response to temptation must be an immediate "No!" The longer we allow temptation to linger in our minds, the more difficult it will be to reject it.

St. Peter warns that the devil is like a roaring lion, on the prowl for victims. "Resist him, firm in your faith, knowing that the same experience of suffering is required of your brotherhood throughout the world" (1 Pet. 5:9).

Temptation, in itself, is not always a bad thing. All of the great saints had to overcome temptation. St. James tells us, "... the testing of your faith produces steadfastness" (Jas. 1:2-3). Even Jesus was "one who in every respect has been tempted as we are, yet without sinning" (Heb. 4:15).

> *He did not say: You will not be assailed, you will not be belabored, you will not be disquieted, but he said: You will not be overcome.*
>
> — BLESSED JULIAN OF NORWICH
>
> ✑

Temptations can strengthen our will, increase our faith and become a means of purification. Temptations help us to recognize our need for God. "Blessed is the man who endures trial, for when he has stood the test he will receive the crown of life which God has promised to those who love him" (Jas. 1:12).

St. Paul assures us that God does not cause us to be tempted, but He allows it to happen, and offers the grace we need to overcome it. "God is faithful and he will not let you be tempted beyond your strength; but with the temptation will also provide the way of escape, that you may be able to endure it" (1 Cor. 10:13).

RESISTING TEMPTATIONS

In the Garden of Gethsemane, Jesus warned His apostles, "Watch and pray that you may not enter into temptation" (Mt. 26:41).

To watch means to know your weaknesses so that you won't be caught off guard by temptations. We all have weaknesses, and it's important to know the areas where you are most likely to waver.

Prayer is also good protection against temptation, because it invites God to come to our aid. We entrust ourselves to His care. Some people invoke the name of Jesus. Some people ask for the intercession of Our Lady and the saints.

St. Teresa of Ávila suggests that we treat temptations with contempt. "Let this be known well, that every time we make them the object of our contempt, they lose their strength and the soul acquires over them greater ascendancy."

Contemporary spiritual writer Henry Nouwen tells us not to be surprised by temptations. "They will increase, but as you face them without fear, you will discover that they are powerless. What is important is to keep clinging to the real, lasting, and unambiguous love of Jesus."

> *Let us ask our Lord to be with us in our moments of temptation. We must not be afraid, because God loves us and will not fail to help us.*
>
> — BLESSED MOTHER TERESA OF CALCUTTA

TALKING ABOUT TEMPTATIONS

It's important to tell someone about your temptations. Your initial reaction may be embarrassment or even feelings of shame, but don't let those feelings stop you from telling a priest or spiritual director what you are experiencing. St. Francis de Sales assures us, "A temptation disclosed is a temptation half-vanquished."

As you become more experienced in recognizing and fighting off temptations, the intensity usually weakens. But there may be special times when temptations will return with full force. Be wary of temptations when you are tired, when you feel weaker than usual, when you are in pain, when you experience uncomfortable side effects from treatments, and when you receive bad news about a recurrence or the spread of your disease to another part of your body. These are the times when you will be most vulnerable.

Sometimes, what seems like a temptation is really part of your illness. If you find yourself sinking into depression or experiencing thoughts of suicide, tell your doctor immediately. The cause of your depression may be related to your treatment and can be alleviated with proper medication.

> *We gain the strength of the temptations we resist.*
>
> — RALPH WALDO EMERSON

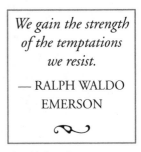

In your fight against temptation, you will discover that your faith is strengthened, and you can proclaim with St. Paul, "If God is for us, who is against us?" (Rom. 8:31).

A good prayer for this stage of your journey invokes the help of St. Michael the Archangel:

St. Michael the Archangel,
defend us in battle.
Be our protection against the wickedness
and snares of the devil.
May God rebuke him, we humbly pray;
and do Thou, O Prince of the Heavenly Host,
by the Divine Power of God,
cast into hell Satan and all the other evil spirits
who roam throughout the world seeking the ruin of souls.

Amen.

QUESTIONS FOR REFLECTION

1. What kinds of temptation have you faced?
2. What techniques do you use to overcome temptation?
3. How has your faith been strengthened because of temptation?

Reaching Out

The first time it happened, I was waiting for a radiation treatment. A woman smiled and asked me what kind of cancer I had. Her question startled me. I always thought doctor's offices and hospitals were places where people didn't talk to one another. But that unspoken rule does not apply to cancer patients. In the next few minutes, she shared her story, and I shared mine. A bond formed. I had been initiated into the community of cancer patients. It wasn't long before I started striking up conversations with other patients in hallways, waiting rooms, and elevators.

Every cancer patient has a story to tell. The greatest gift we can give another cancer patient is to listen. We listen to their pain, their joys, their struggles, their successes, and their failures. We hear about their families, their friends, their doctors, their treatments.

Before long, we discover that the individual stories become "our" story.

Find out how much God has given you and from it take what you need; the remainder is needed by others.

— ST. AUGUSTINE

The late Cardinal Joseph Bernardin called this phenomenon "a special solidarity" that exists between cancer patients. He saw his involvement with other cancer patients as a special cancer ministry. His treatments took only ten minutes, but his hospital visits sometimes lasted as long as five hours, as he talked and prayed with people. He compiled a long prayer list with the names of other patients and their families.

"Time and again I have stood in awe as people suffering from life-threatening illnesses have shared with me their insights into life," he recalled. "I have been inspired to see how truly human and how truly wise they are. So often in the past, I, like most of us, have struggled with what to say to people who are suffering. But since I was diagnosed as having cancer, words come more easily. So has the ability to know when to listen or simply reach out my hand."

NEW LESSONS LEARNED

Reaching out to others gives new meaning to your life and to your experience of cancer. In the process you learn some new things about yourself.

- You become more understanding — not just of others, but also of yourself and your own situation.
- You become more compassionate. In fact, the word "compassion" comes from the Latin words that mean "to suffer with."
- You become more patient. St. Augustine tells us, "Patience is the companion of wisdom."
- You become less self-centered. You begin to see your situation in relation to everyone who has cancer. You become part of the whole.
- You discover that the real essence of life is our ability to love God and our neighbor. Jesus assures us that when you understand this, "You are not far from the kingdom of God" (Mk. 12:28-34).

The late Cardinal Basil Hume once said, "I see this life as a period of training, a time of preparation, during which we learn the art of loving God and our neighbor."

If you turn to your Catholic faith, you will see that Jesus encourages us to treat others as we would like to be treated (Mt. 7:12). He also assures us that whatever we do for our brothers and sisters, we do for Him (Mt. 25:40).

You don't even have to worry about what to say to another person because Jesus promises: ". . . what you are to say will be given to you in that hour; for it is not you who speak, but the Spirit of your Father speaking through you" (Mt. 10:19-20).

REACHING OUT IN BIGGER WAYS

Sometimes, reaching out to others goes beyond one-to-one conversations. Stories abound of people, inspired by their experience of cancer, who go on to do extraordinary things.

- They start prayer groups, support groups, and cancer ministries.
- They start foundations and organize fundraising events for cancer research.
- They give inspirational talks about how cancer has impacted their lives.
- They develop new programs to create awareness of cancer prevention.
- They serve as volunteers in cancer hospitals and clinics.
- They find creative ways of helping other people in their fight against this devastating disease.

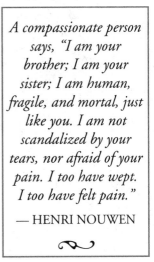

A compassionate person says, "I am your brother; I am your sister; I am human, fragile, and mortal, just like you. I am not scandalized by your tears, nor afraid of your pain. I too have wept. I too have felt pain."

— HENRI NOUWEN

By reaching out to others, you become what Henri Nouwen calls "a wounded healer." A wounded healer is someone who uses his or her own painful experience to become a source of new life for others. Nouwen insists that the deepest motivation for reaching out to others springs from hope. "For hope makes it possible to look beyond the fulfillment of urgent wishes and pressing desires and offers a vision beyond human suffering and even death.... Hope prevents us from clinging to what we have and frees us to move away from the safe place and enter unknown and fearful territory.... It is an act of discipleship in which we follow the hard road of Christ, who entered death with nothing but bare hope."

The perfect prayer at this stage of the journey is the Prayer of St. Francis:

Lord, make me an instrument of Your peace.
Where there is hatred, let me sow love;
where there is injury, pardon;
where there is doubt, faith;

where there is despair, hope;
where there is darkness, light;
and where there is sadness, joy.

O Divine Master,
grant that I may not so much seek
to be consoled as to console;
to be understood as to understand;
to be loved as to love;
for it is in giving that we receive;
it is in pardoning that we are pardoned;
and it is in dying that we are born to eternal life.

∾ QUESTIONS FOR REFLECTION ∾

1. In what ways have other cancer patients reached out to you?
2. How have you reached out to others?
3. What have you learned from your experience of reaching out?

Finding Inner Peace

*E*arly in my treatment for breast cancer, I remember asking my doctor when my life would go back to normal. He paused, then replied, "Don't think of it as going back to where you were before. Even if you didn't have cancer, you wouldn't be the same person a year or two from now that you are today. Think of yourself as continuing on a journey through life."

It was the best advice he could have given me. I stopped looking back and I stopped fearing the future. In the process, I began to discover the presence of God in the most ordinary places.

- I felt God's presence whenever a volunteer at the cancer hospital opened the door and wished me a good day.
- I felt God's presence when a friend offered to take me to a doctor's appointment.
- I felt God's presence during radiation treatments as I imagined His healing love destroying my cancer cells.
- I felt God's presence every time I watered the plants or fed the goldfish that came to me as "get well" presents.
- I felt God's presence when I woke up in the morning and when I went to bed at night.

> *Be at peace with your own soul, then heaven and earth will be at peace with you.*
>
> — ST. JEROME
>
> ~

I knew from my Catholic faith that God is everywhere, but I had never had the ability to see so clearly with eyes of faith. It made every day a new adventure. Where would I see God today? What little miracles would I encounter?

FEELING GRATEFUL

I'd often heard the cliché "vicious cycle" to describe things going from bad to worse. In some strange way, what I experienced was a "grace-filled cycle," where every experience of God led me to a deeper sense of joy. Even in the midst of pain, if I could see or feel the presence of God, the result was an overwhelming sense of gratitude.

Cancer gave me the opportunity to appreciate each minute of every day, to be grateful for family members and friends, to look back on the joys of my life, to enjoy little things in life, to focus on the important things and let go of the unimportant.

I found myself being grateful for small acts of kindness from doctors, nurses, technicians, volunteers, and strangers. My prayer at this stage of the journey became, "Thank you, Lord, for what you are teaching me in this experience of having cancer."

I even found myself telling other people, "I never would have asked for cancer, but I'm not sorry that I've experienced this, because it changed me in ways I never anticipated."

... give thanks in all circumstances, for this is the will of God in Christ Jesus for you.

— 1 THESS. 5:18

A NEW LIFE

The experience of cancer can become a process of spiritual transformation, in which you discover a new sense of meaning and purpose. You develop a new outlook on life and a new way of living. Your old life is gone, and a new life has begun. You discover your true self. You find a deep sense of inner peace.

Another cancer patient summed it up when she recalled the day she sat at the kitchen table looking at old photos of herself before her diagnosis of cancer. She was stunned when she remembered how shallow and superficial her life had been before cancer. She hadn't asked the deep questions or penetrated the surface of her being. She hadn't discovered the depths of her own spiritual life. She hadn't had the chance to move outside of herself and help other people. Her life had been focused on material things. She hadn't discovered that penetrating sense of peace that only God can instill.

"I like you better now," her son told her.

Like the grain of wheat that Jesus talks about in the Gospels, her old life ended, but a new life began and it was already bearing good fruit (Jn.12:24).

We know that in everything God works for good with those who love him ...

— ROM. 8:28

THE GIFT OF PEACE

Two weeks before Cardinal Joseph Bernardin died from pancreatic cancer, he wrote: "What I would like to leave behind is a simple prayer that each of you may find what I have found — God's special gift to us all: the gift of peace. When we are at peace, we find the freedom to be most fully who we are, even in the worst of times."

Bishop Fulton Sheen described this deep inner peace as being "like the great ocean whose bosom is always sighing and heaving in restlessness, but whose great depths are calm and unshaken."

It is the peace that Jesus promised when He said, "Peace I leave with you; my peace I give to you; not as the world gives do I give to you" (Jn.14:27).

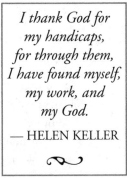

I thank God for my handicaps, for through them, I have found myself, my work, and my God.

— HELEN KELLER

It is the same deep peace in St. Paul's assurance that "the peace of God, which passes all understanding, will keep your hearts and your minds in Christ Jesus" (Phil. 4:7).

It is the same peace that St. Thérèse of Lisieux described when she was told that she had only a month to live. "I will not fear, for God will give me strength; He'll never abandon me."

THE POWER OF PEACE

I wish that I could end this book like a fairy tale, with the assurance that everyone will live happily ever after, but that would be unrealistic. I can, however, offer you the assurance that it is possible to live peacefully ever after — no matter what happens.

A year after I was diagnosed with breast cancer, I began the journey all over again when I was diagnosed with uterine cancer. I found myself going back through each of the spiritual milestones, skipping more quickly past some and pausing for a longer period of time at others. But the second time around was different, because I carried within me a deep sense of peace.

It was the same deep sense of peace that sustained me a few months later when Michael, my daughter's 26-year-old boyfriend, died from malignant melanoma.

There are no guarantees with cancer. Even if you are cured of cancer or in remission, there will be times when you may begin to feel anxious about an upcoming checkup or fearful that your cancer has returned. You can rely on that deep sense of peace to sustain you.

Even if you are told that you will die from cancer, if you can place your trust in God, that deep sense of peace will sustain you. Peace will come to you when you find meaning in life — whether that life will last ten more days, ten more months, or ten more years.

A friend told me the story of a Canadian woman whose treatments were not working. Her doctors said she only had a short time to live. She immediately asked all of her family and friends to stop praying for her recovery, and instead, to send her whatever intentions they wanted her to present to God when she died. Word spread, and within a month she had received more than 1,000 prayer requests. It gave her life meaning and hope to the very end.

A wonderful prayer — and a great source of peace for the rest of your journey — is the Prayer of St. Francis de Sales:

Do not look forward in fear to the changes of life;

Rather look to them with full hope that as they arise, God, whose very own you are, will lead you safely through all things;

And when you cannot stand it, God will carry you in His arms.

Do not fear what may happen tomorrow;

The same everlasting Father who cares for you today will take care of you today and every day.

He will either shield you from suffering or will give you unfailing strength to bear it.

Be at peace and put aside all anxious thoughts and imaginations.

ᗏ QUESTIONS FOR REFLECTION ᘒ

1. In what ways have you felt the presence of God on your journey through cancer?
2. What are you grateful for?
3. How would you describe your sense of inner peace?

Resources

*M*any parishes offer cancer ministries that provide hope, emotional and spiritual support, and resources to cancer patients, their families, and their friends.

Catholic hospitals also sponsor support groups where you can share the daily challenges and ease the stress of cancer diagnosis and treatment with others.

BOOKS

Bernardin, Joseph Cardinal, *The Gift of Peace*. Chicago, IL: Loyola Press, 1997.

Lewis, C. S., *The Problem of Pain*. New York, NY: Simon and Schuster Inc., 1996.

Neuhaus, Richard John, *As I Lay Dying*. New York, NY: Basic Books, 2002.

Nouwen, Henri J., *The Wounded Healer*. New York, NY: Doubleday, 1972.

O'Malley, Vincent J., *Ordinary Suffering of Extraordinary Saints*. Huntington, IN: Our Sunday Visitor, 2000.

Willig, Jim, with Tammy Bundy, *Lessons from the School of Suffering*. Cincinnati, OH: St. Anthony Messenger Press, 2001.

WEB SITES

National Cancer Institute:
www.nci.nih.gov/cancertopics/pdq/supportivecare/spirituality/patient

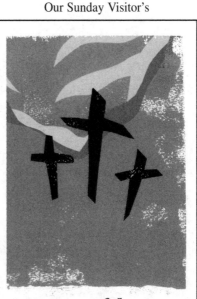

Our Sunday Visitor ...
Your Source for Discovering the Riches of the Catholic Faith

Our Sunday Visitor has an extensive line of materials for young children, teens, and adults. Our books, Bibles, pamphlets, CD-ROMs, audios, and videos are available in bookstores worldwide.

To receive a FREE full-line catalog or for more information, call **Our Sunday Visitor** at **1-800-348-2440, ext. 3**. Or write **Our Sunday Visitor** / 200 Noll Plaza / Huntington, IN 46750.

Please send me ___ A catalog
Please send me materials on:
___ Apologetics and catechetics
___ Prayer books
___ The family
___ Reference works
___ Heritage and the saints
___ The parish

Name _____
Address _____ Apt._____
City _____ State _____ Zip_____
Telephone (   ) _____

A59BBBBP

Please send a friend ___ A catalog
Please send a friend materials on:
___ Apologetics and catechetics
___ Prayer books
___ The family
___ Reference works
___ Heritage and the saints
___ The parish

Name _____
Address _____ Apt._____
City _____ State _____ Zip_____
Telephone (   ) _____

A59BBBBP

OurSundayVisitor

200 Noll Plaza, Huntington, IN 46750
Toll free: **1-800-348-2440**
Website: www.osv.com